The ABCs of DIABETES for Children

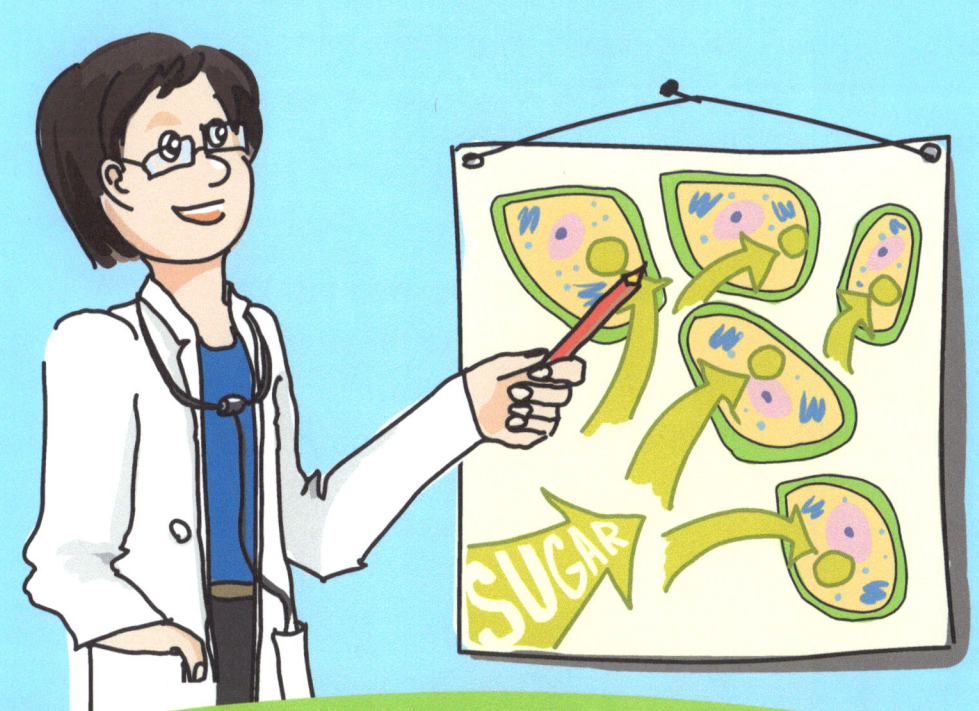

AMANDA JONES

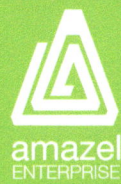

amazel
ENTERPRISE

©2016 by Amazel Enterprise. All rights reserved

All rights reserved. No part of this book may be reproduced or transmitted in any form or by any means, electronic or mechanical, including photocopying, recording, or by an information storage and retrieval system - except by a reviewer who may quote brief passages in a review to be printed in a magazine or newspaper - without permission in writing from the publisher.

Although every precaution has been taken to verify the accuracy of the information contained herein, the author and publisher assume no responsibility for any errors or omissions. No liability is assumed for damages that may result from the use of information contained within

ISBN: 9781707690572

INTRODUCTION

This book aims to create a better understanding of Diabetes for children. It is an educational tool which seeks to bring about change in the approach taken to managing this condition. Echoing the words of Nelson Mandela, Amanda also believes that "education is the most powerful weapon which you can use to change the world." With diabetes children can still run, skip, swim and play.

Book Cover & Layout: bookcoverdeals.com
Publisher: Amazel Enterprise

The body needs ENERGY,
For it to work properly.

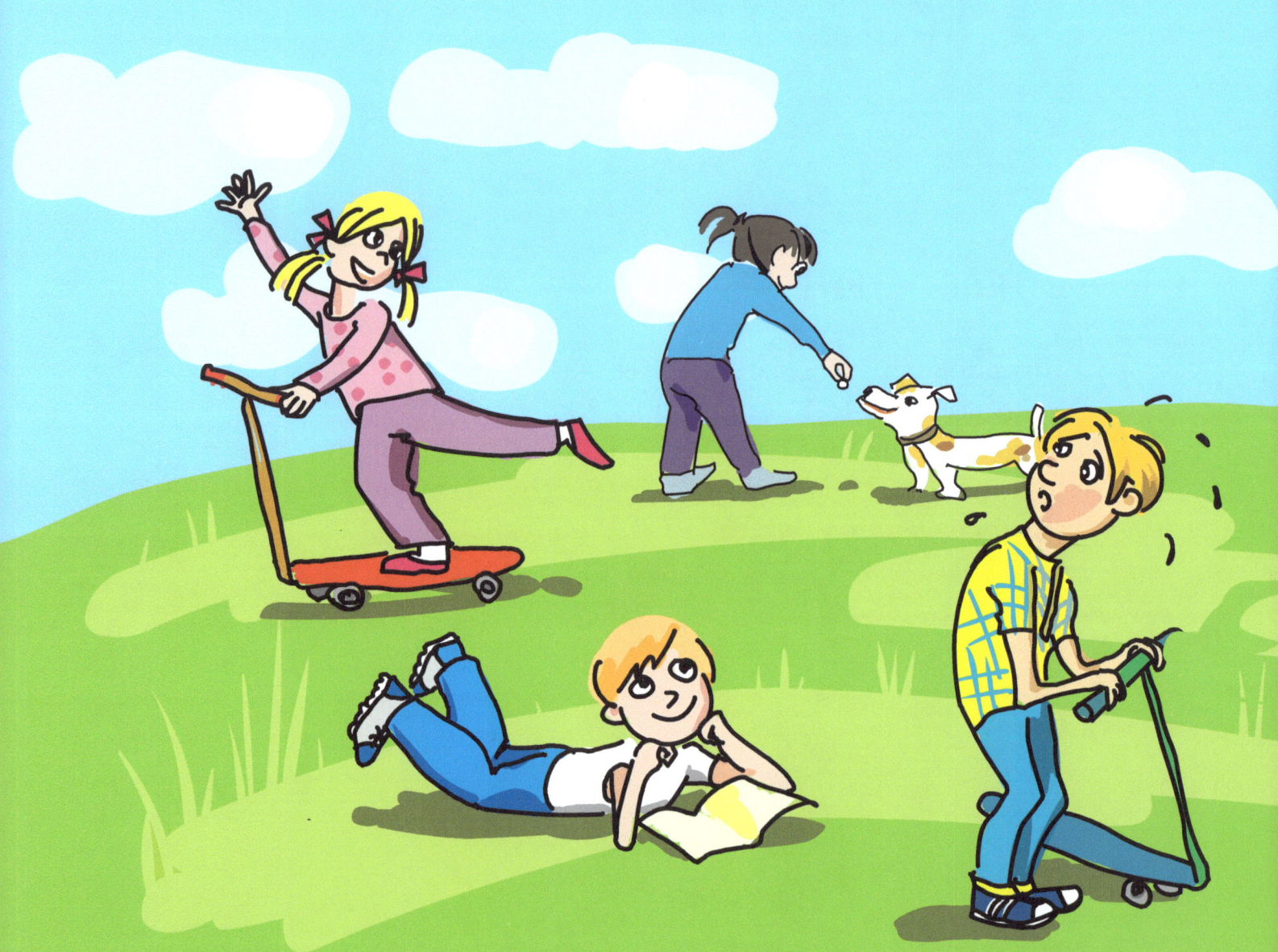

To RUN, SKIP, SWIM or PLAY,
All the time, every single day.

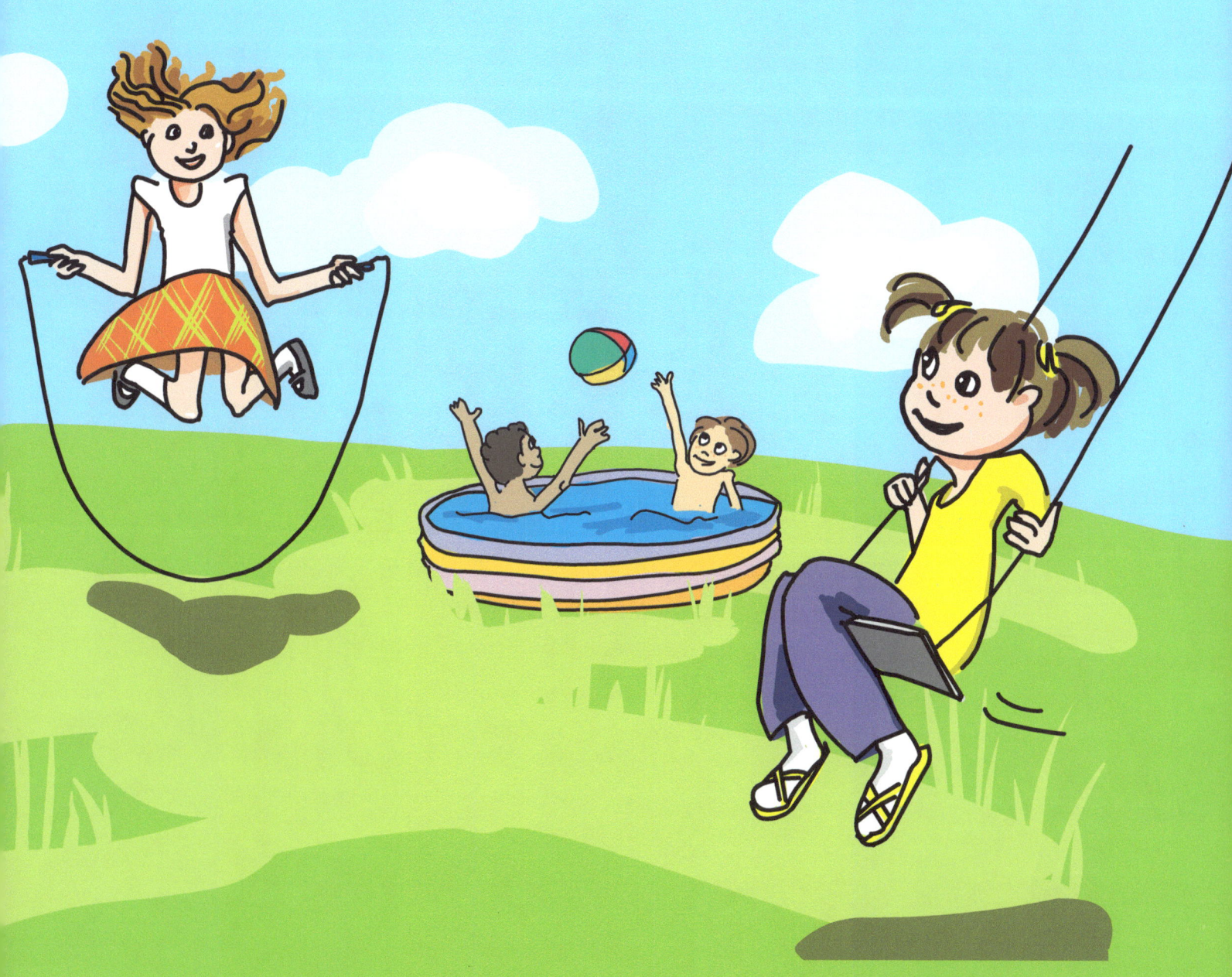

SUGAR gives the energy needed by the body.
It is found in the FOOD that is eaten
and goes into the tummy.

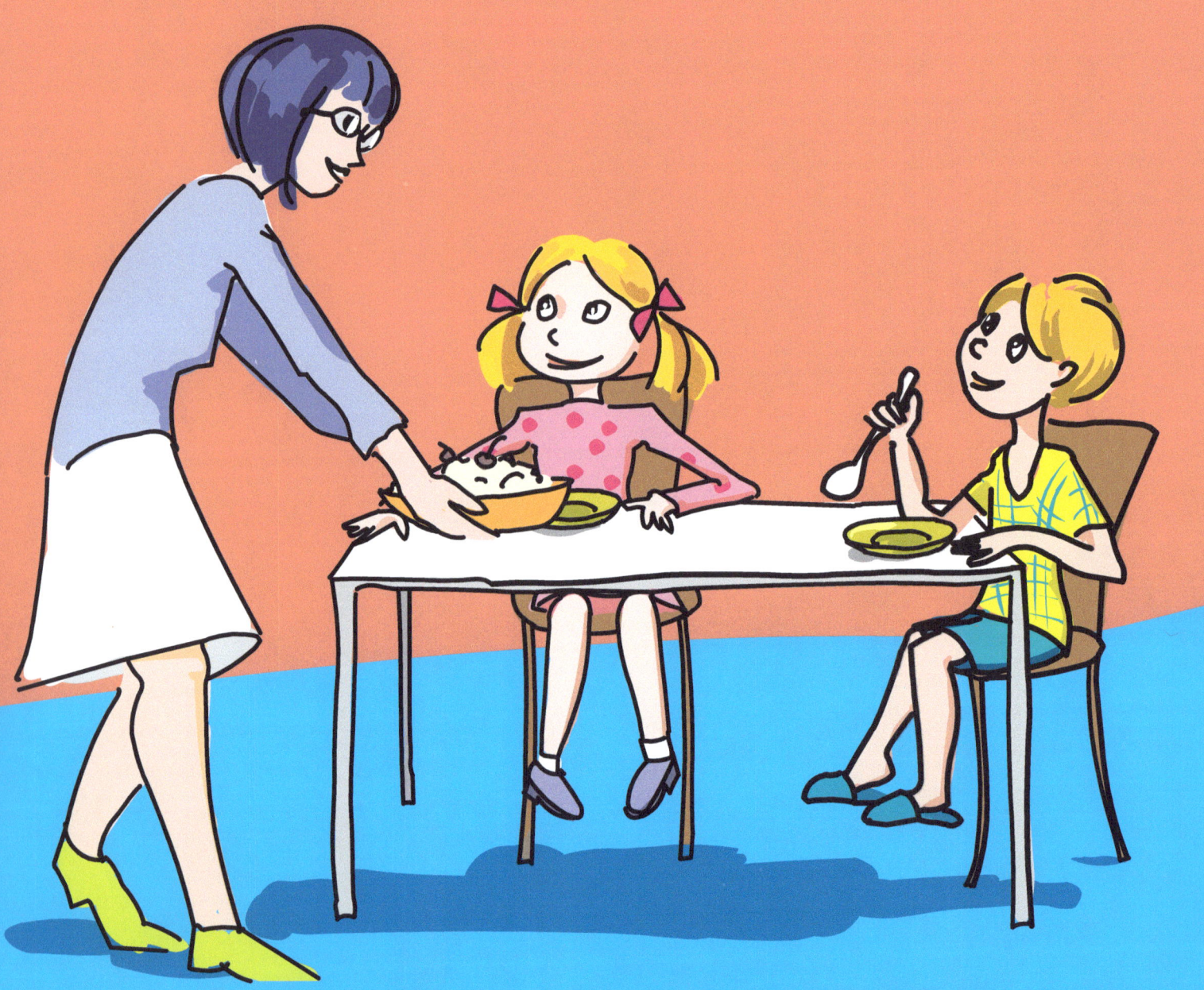

For sugar to do its job well,
It must get into the body's cell.

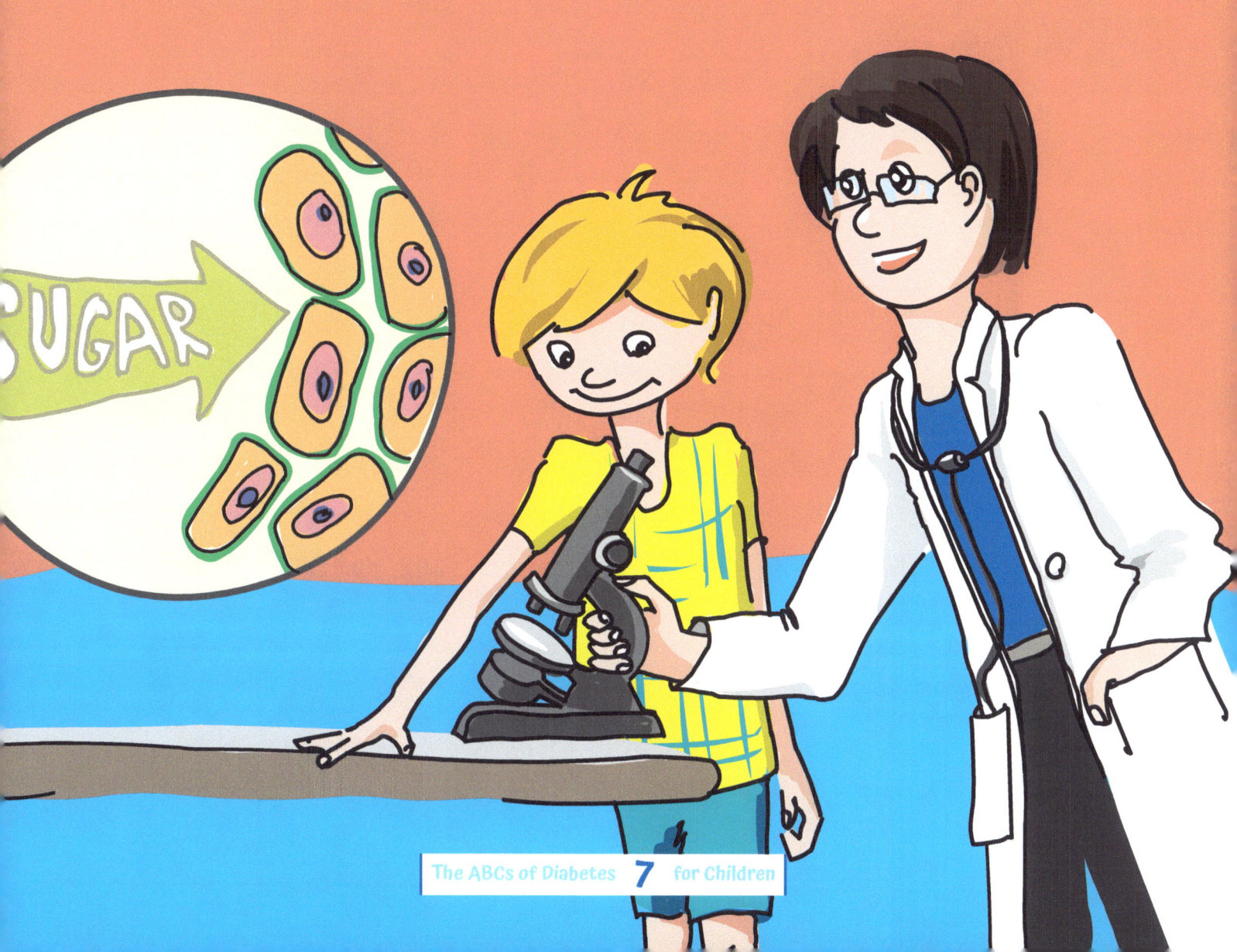

Each CELL has a door which is locked,
And it won't open with just a knock.

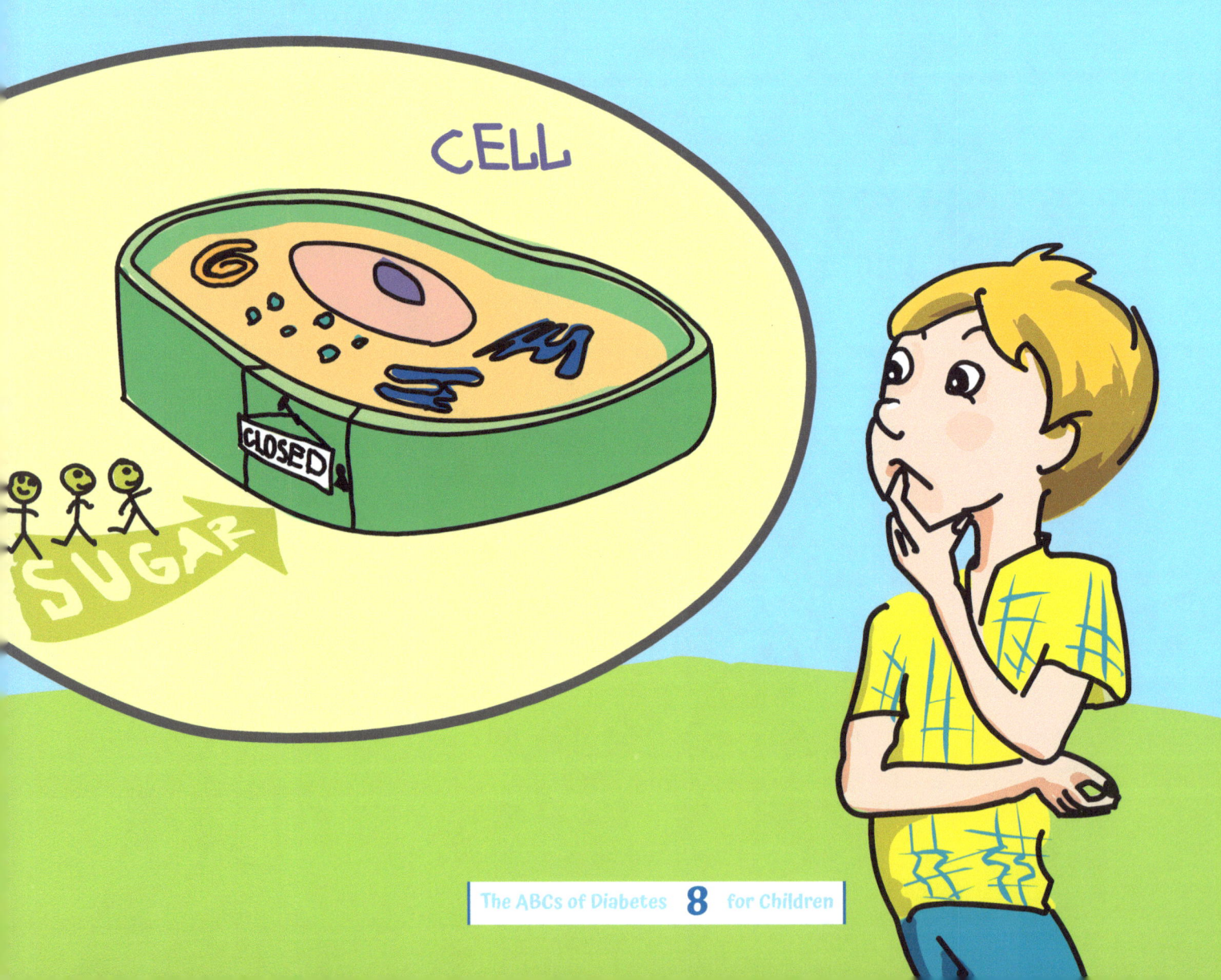

A KEY is needed to open the door and get in,
So the PANCREAS sends keys called INSULIN.

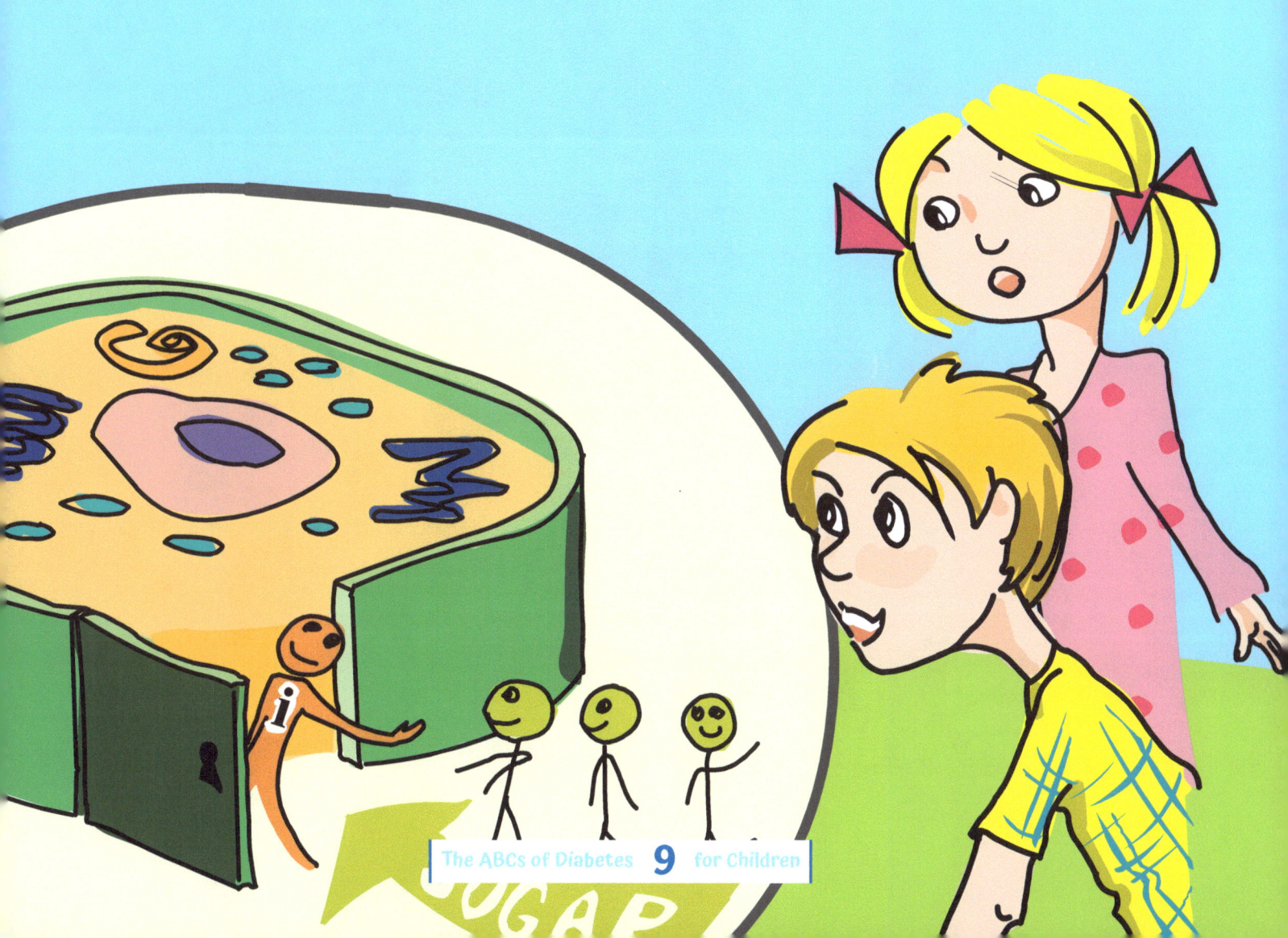

Once the door is open sugar leaves the blood to do its deed,
Of giving the body the energy which it needs.

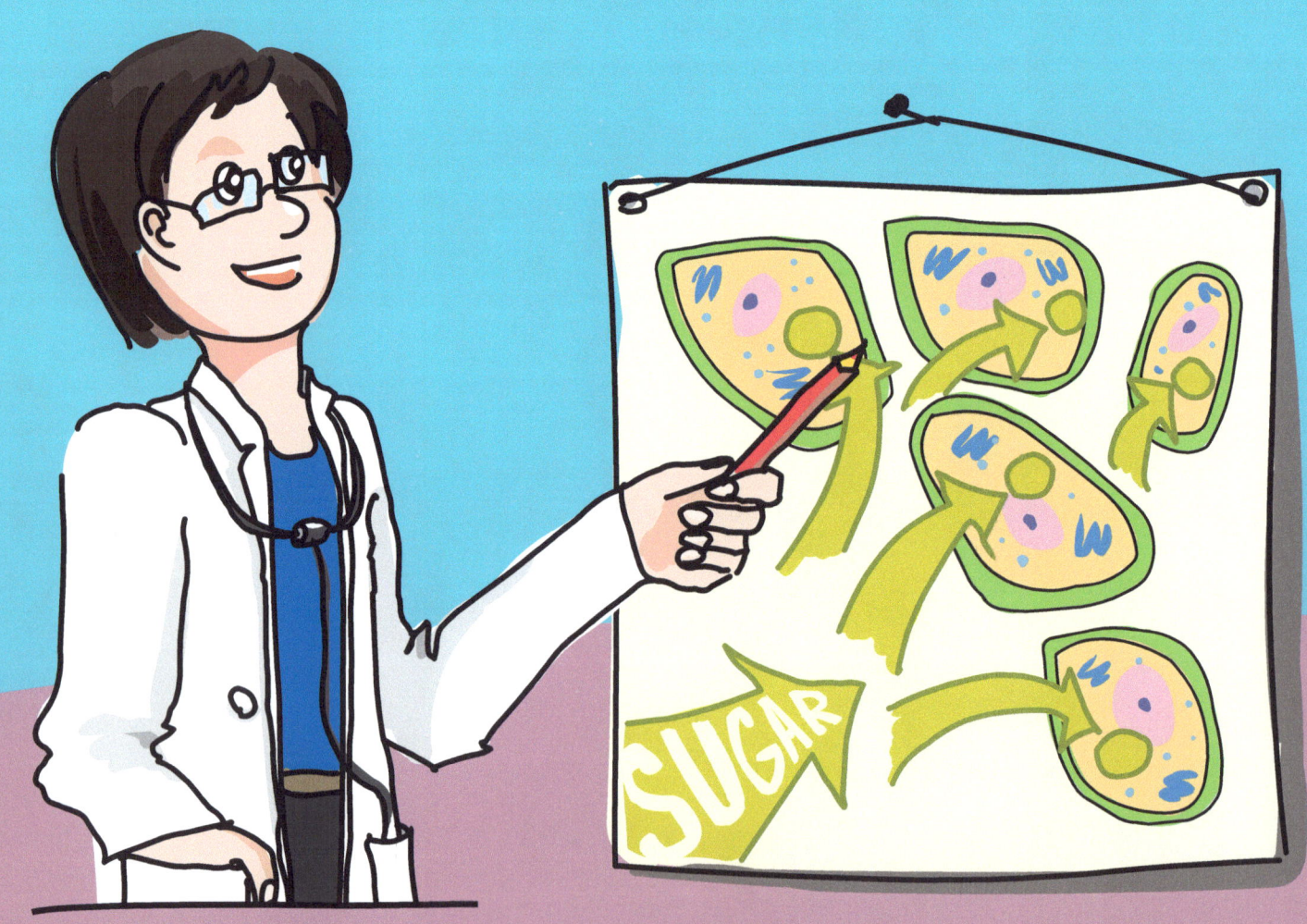

Sometimes the insulin keys may not be enough,
Which makes getting sugar into the cells very tough.

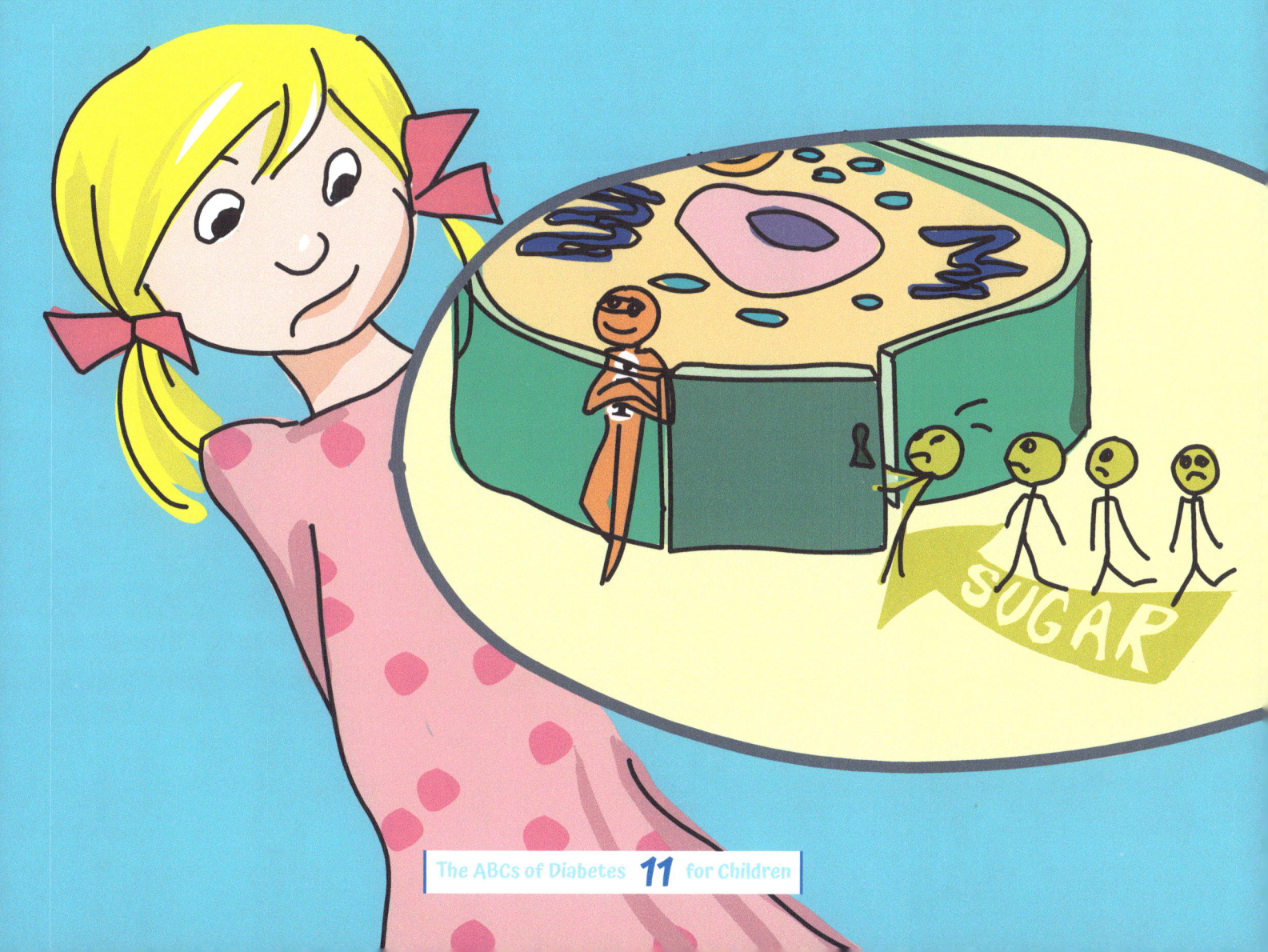

Also, some insulin keys may not open the door,
So sugar's chances of getting into the cells are very poor.

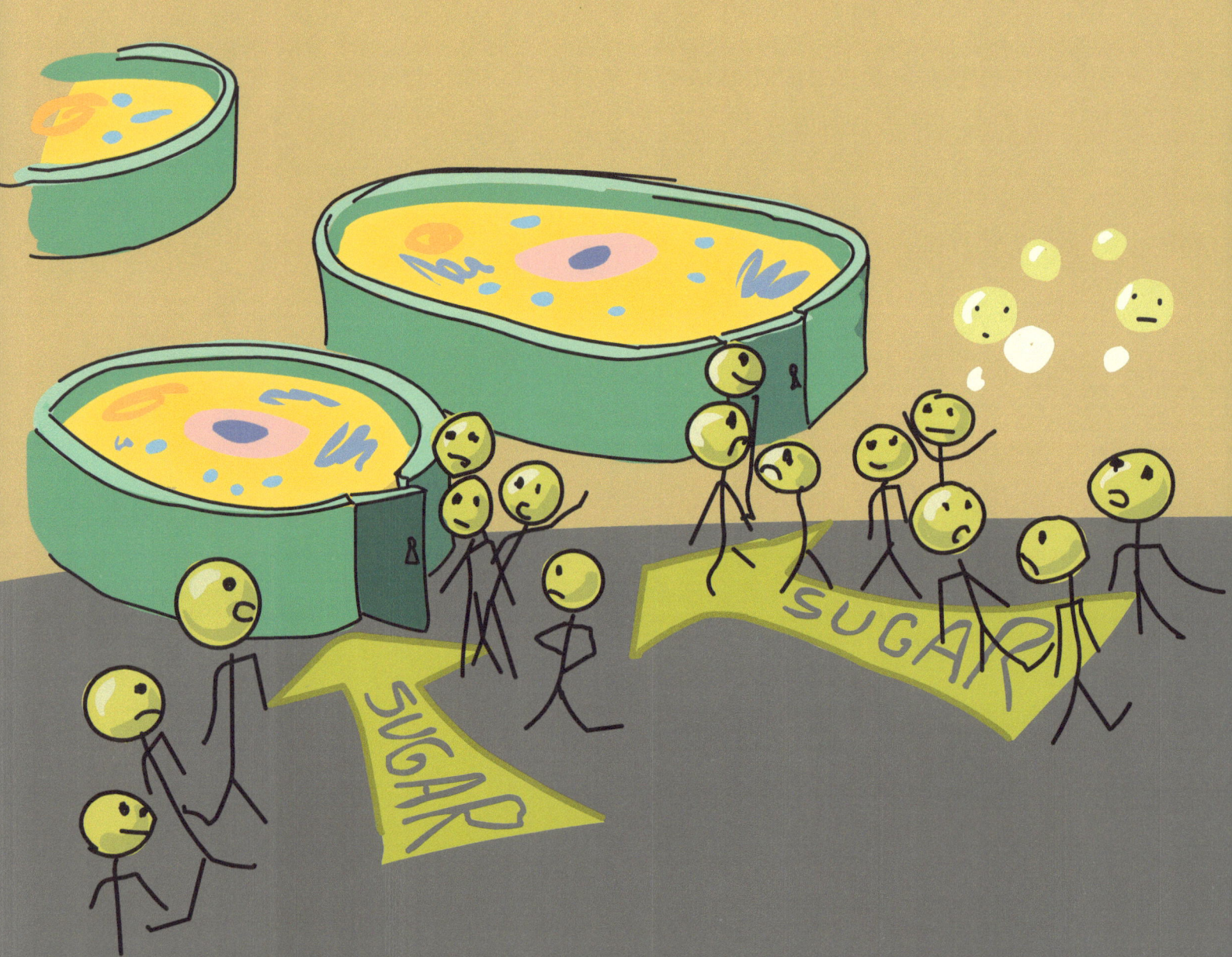

With no entry, sugar stays in the blood, builds up and rise,
Giving the body a DIABETES surprise.

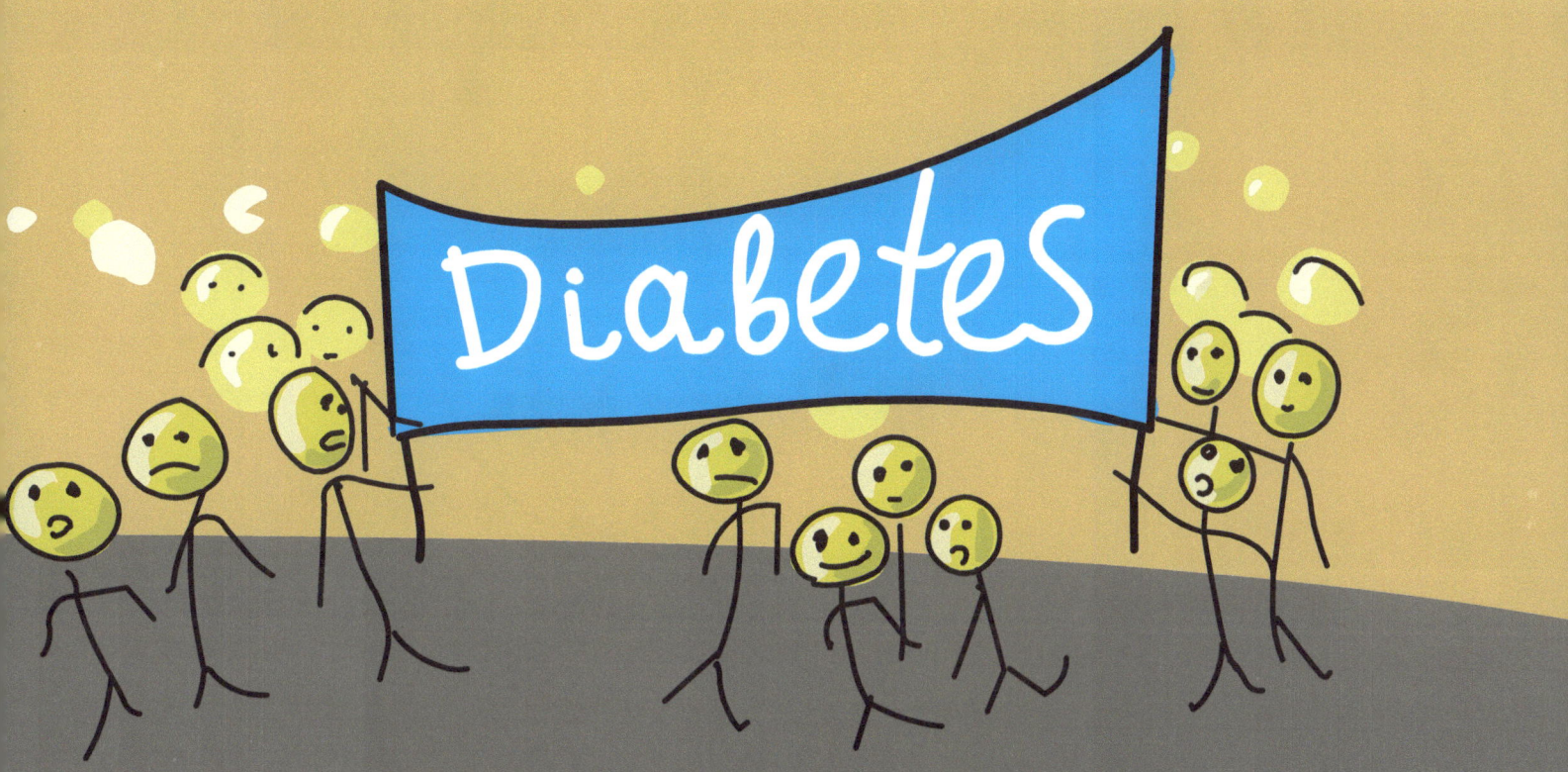

Children are affected by Type 1 usually,
So sometimes from a tender age begins their
DIABETES journey.

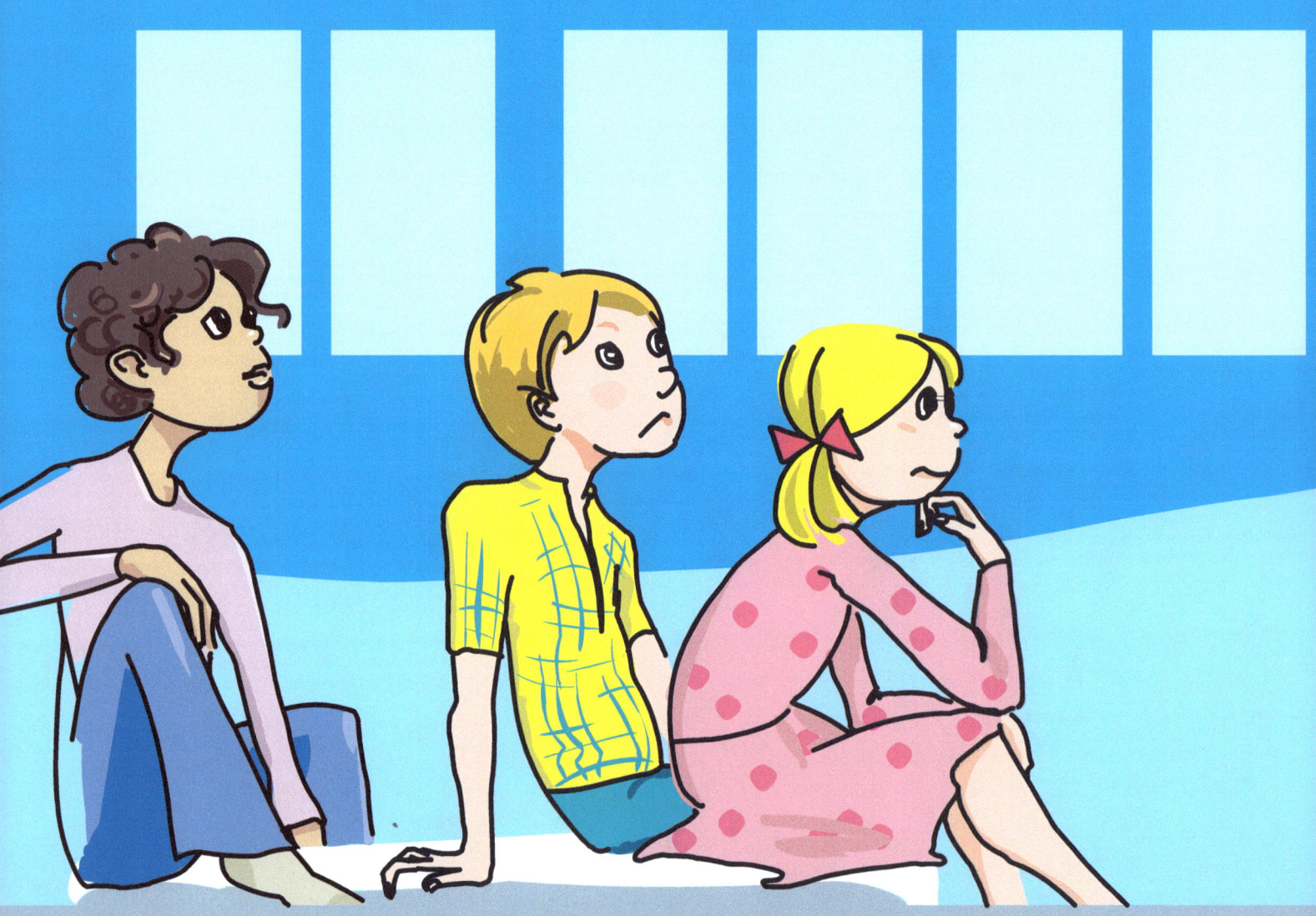

There are signs which will let you know,
That DIABETES may be planning to make a show.

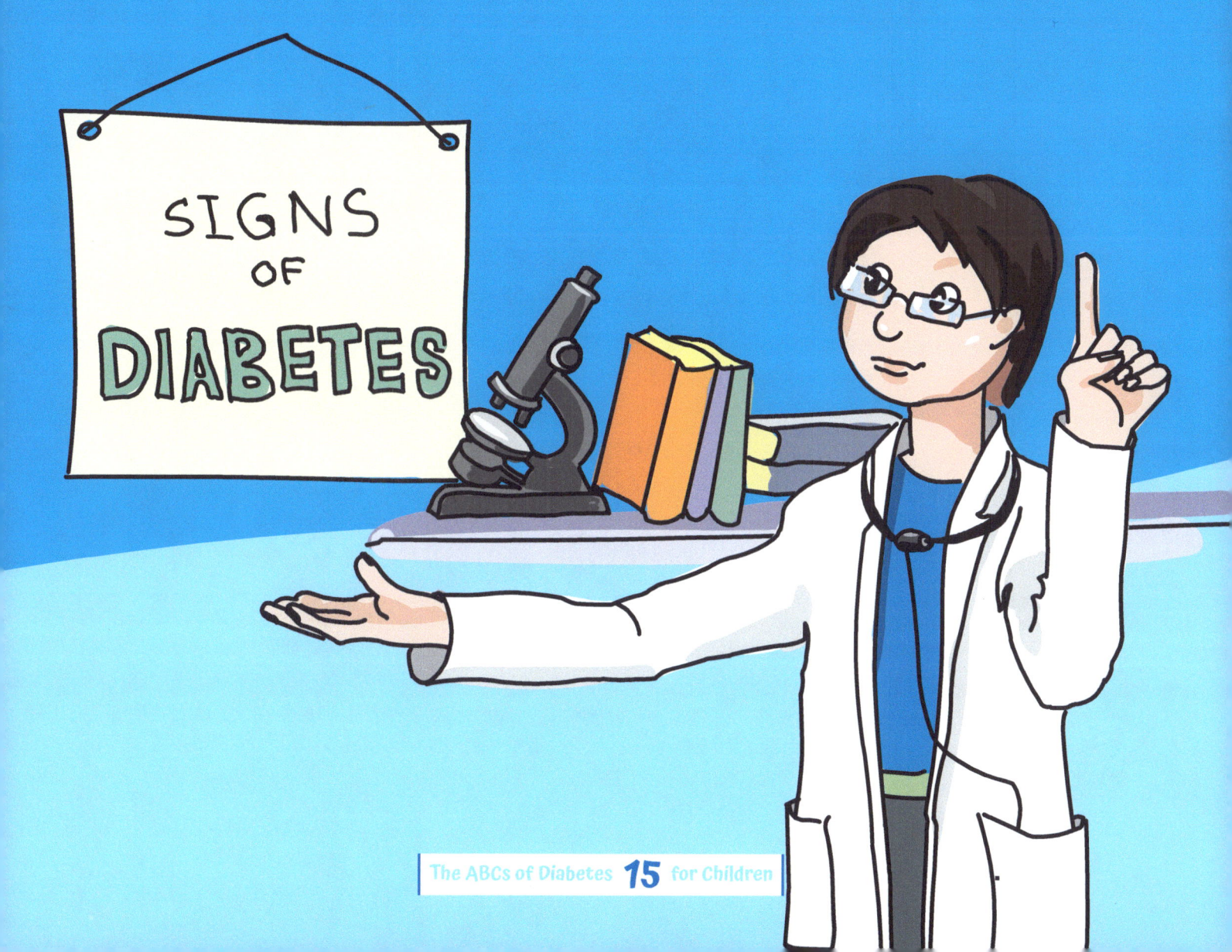

If you often feel TIRED, HUNGRY or THIRSTY,
Have BLURRED EYESIGHT or PASS URINE FREQUENTLY.

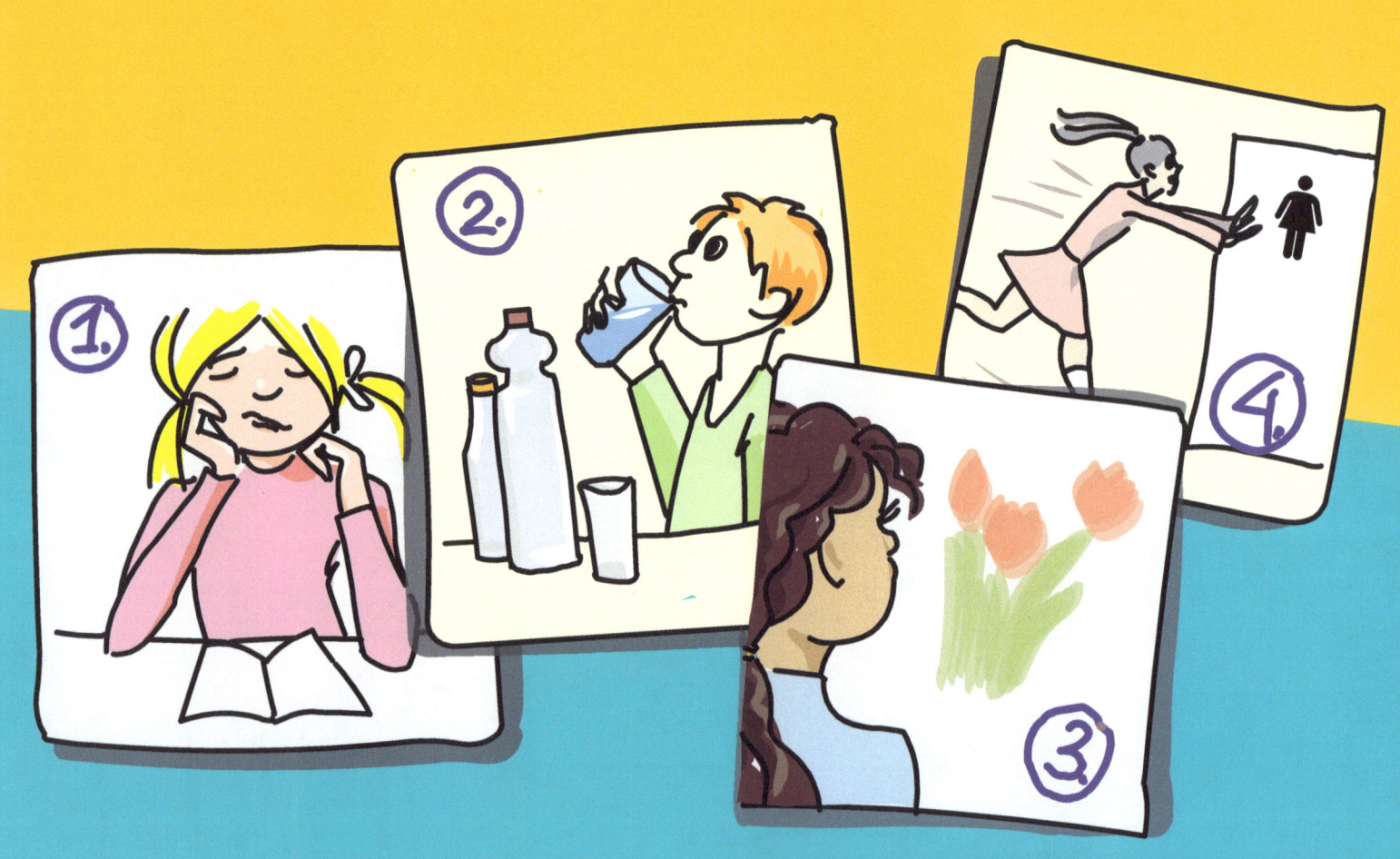

Your parents should take you to the doctor as soon as they can,
To put together a DIABETES fighting plan.

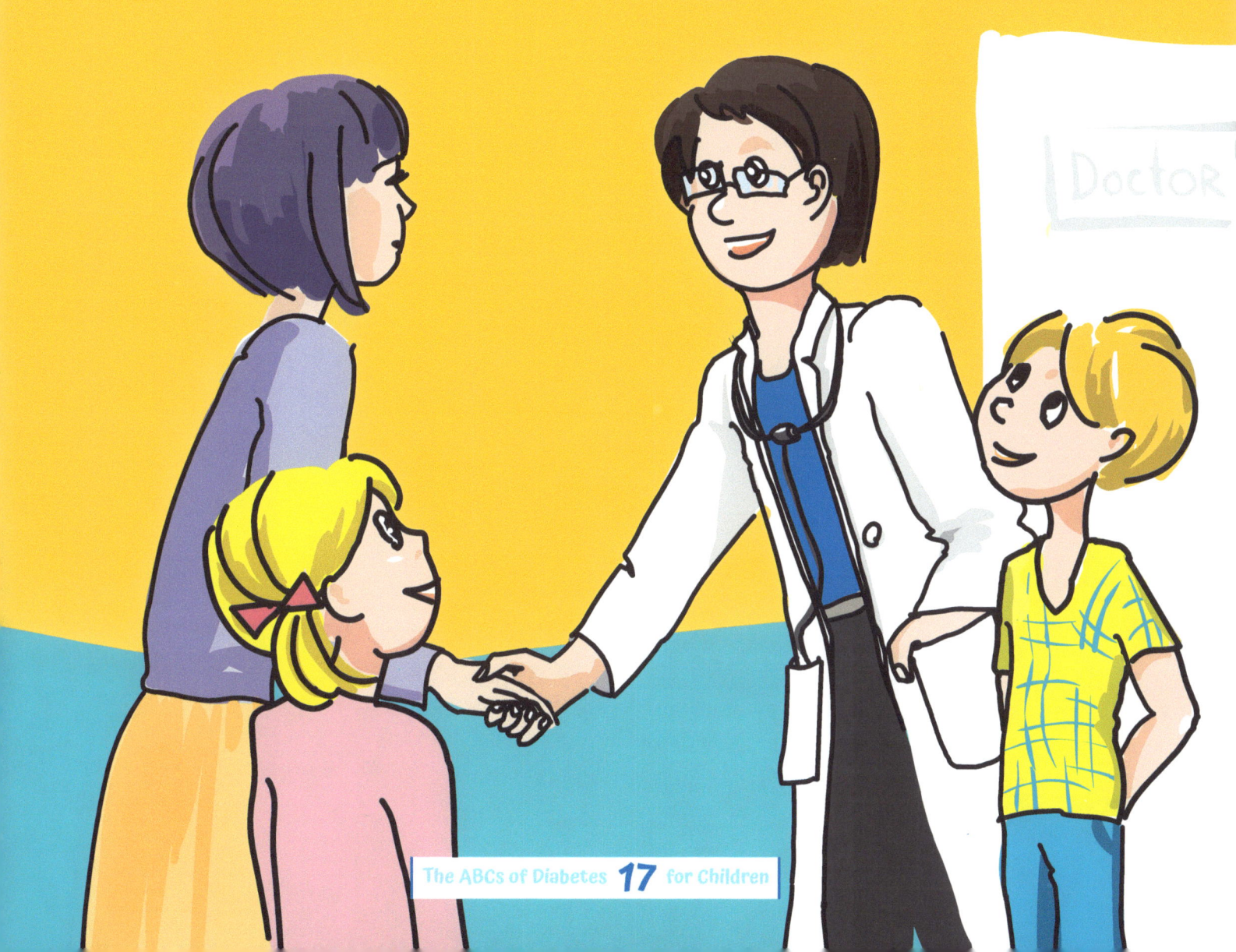

If DIABETES is not taken care of properly,
It can cause harm to different parts of the body.

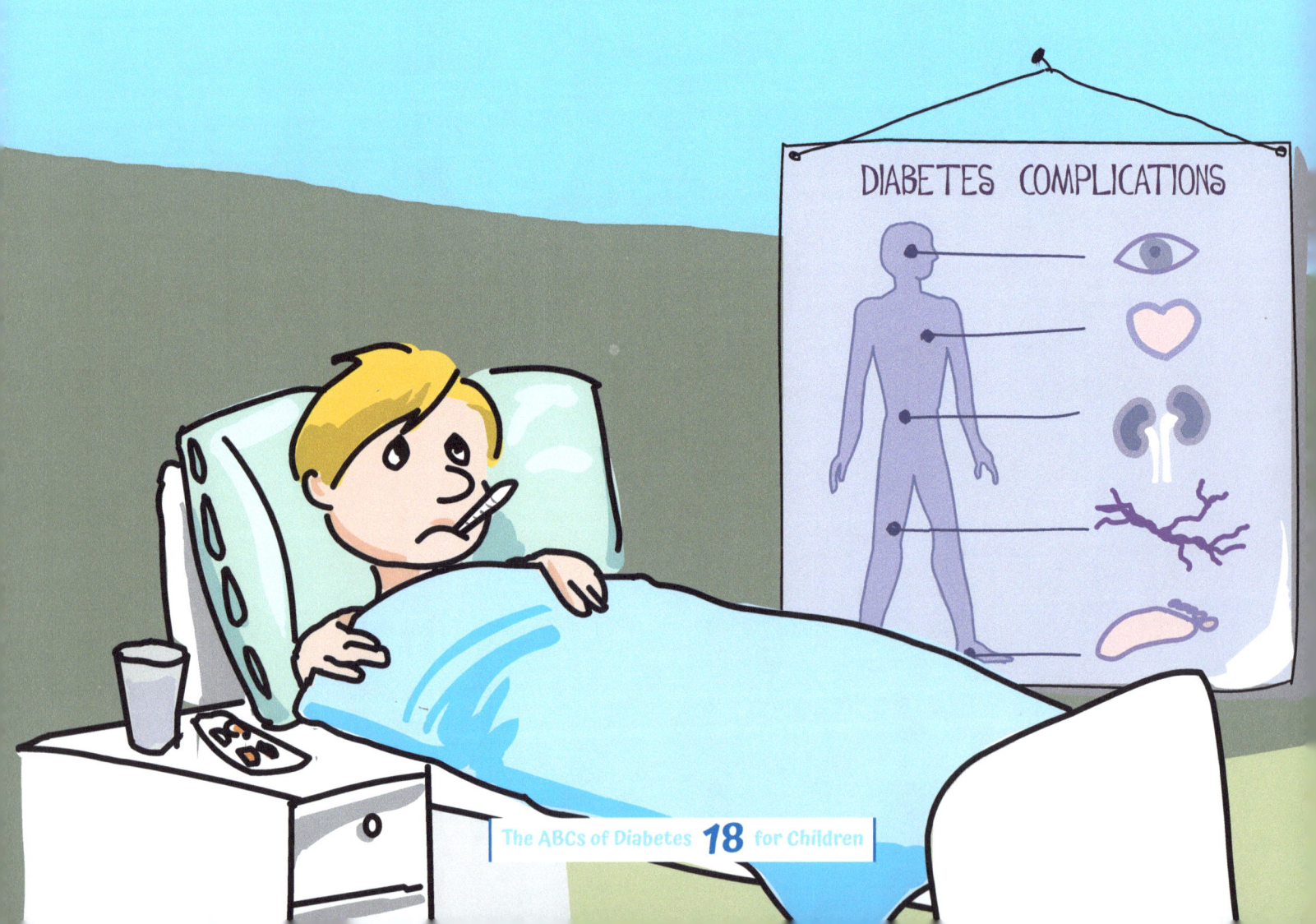

Every one will have to work together, That's you, your parents and the doctor.

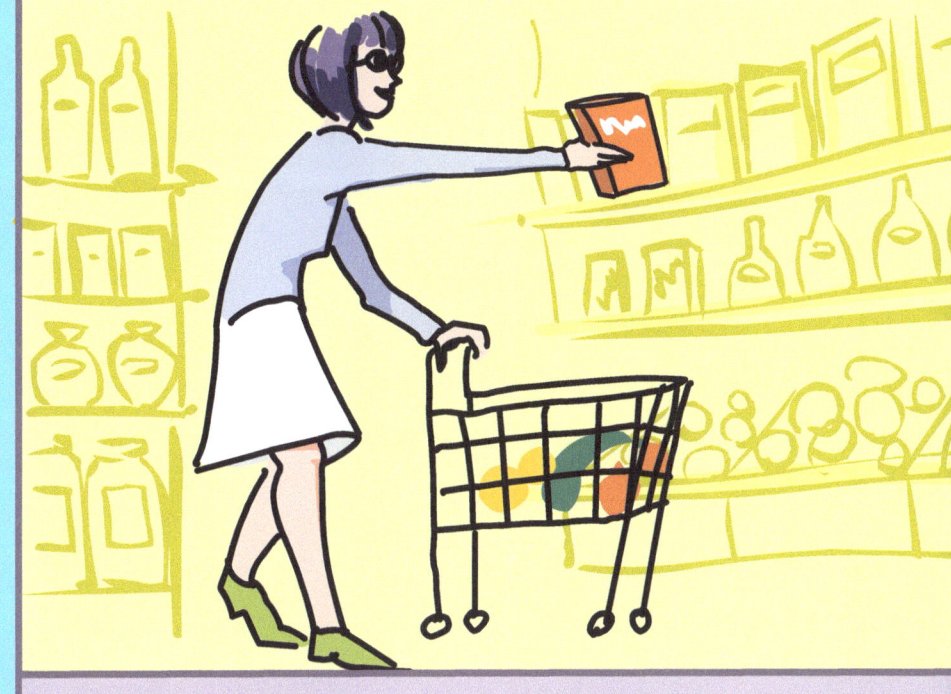
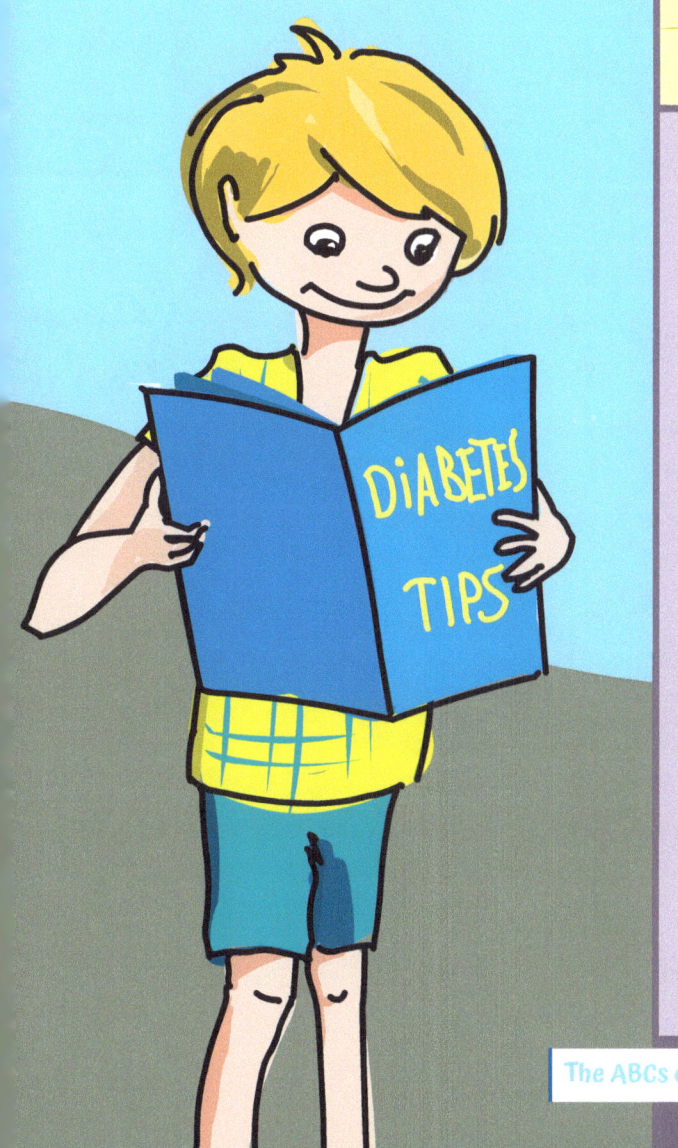
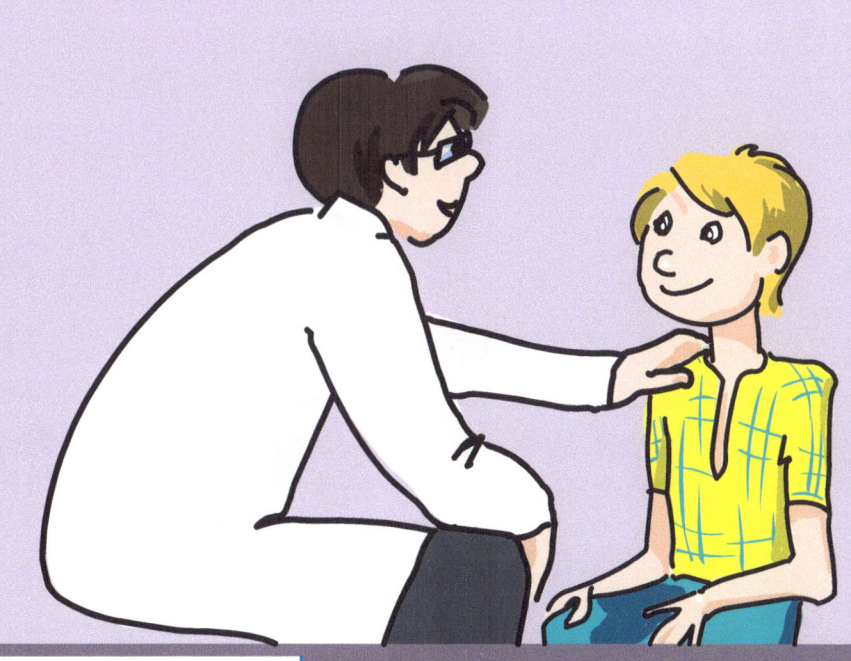

The food eaten should be HEALTHY,
More FRUITS and VEGETABLES...
and less candy.

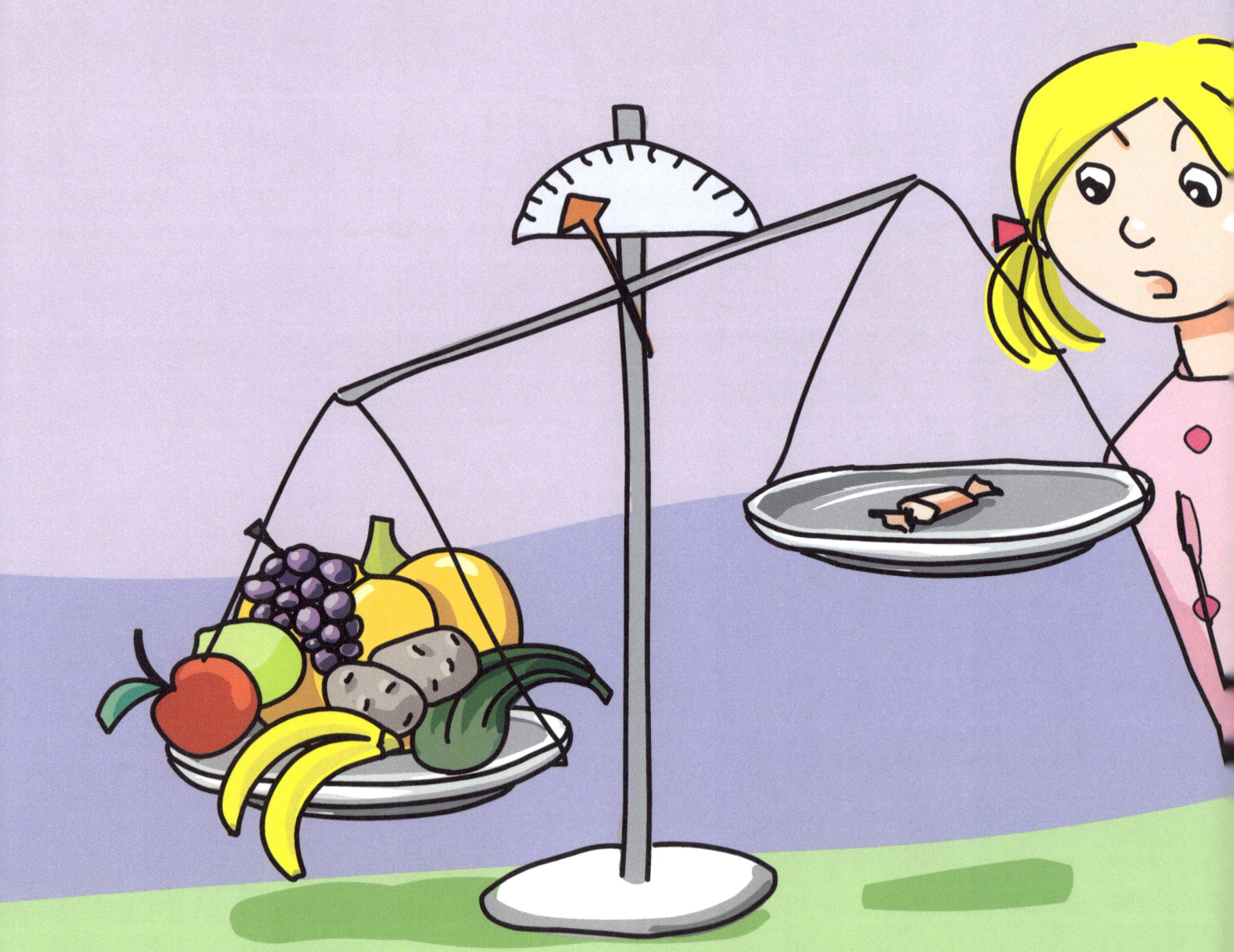

Every day should include a bit of EXERCISE,
To help keep away that DIABETES surprise.

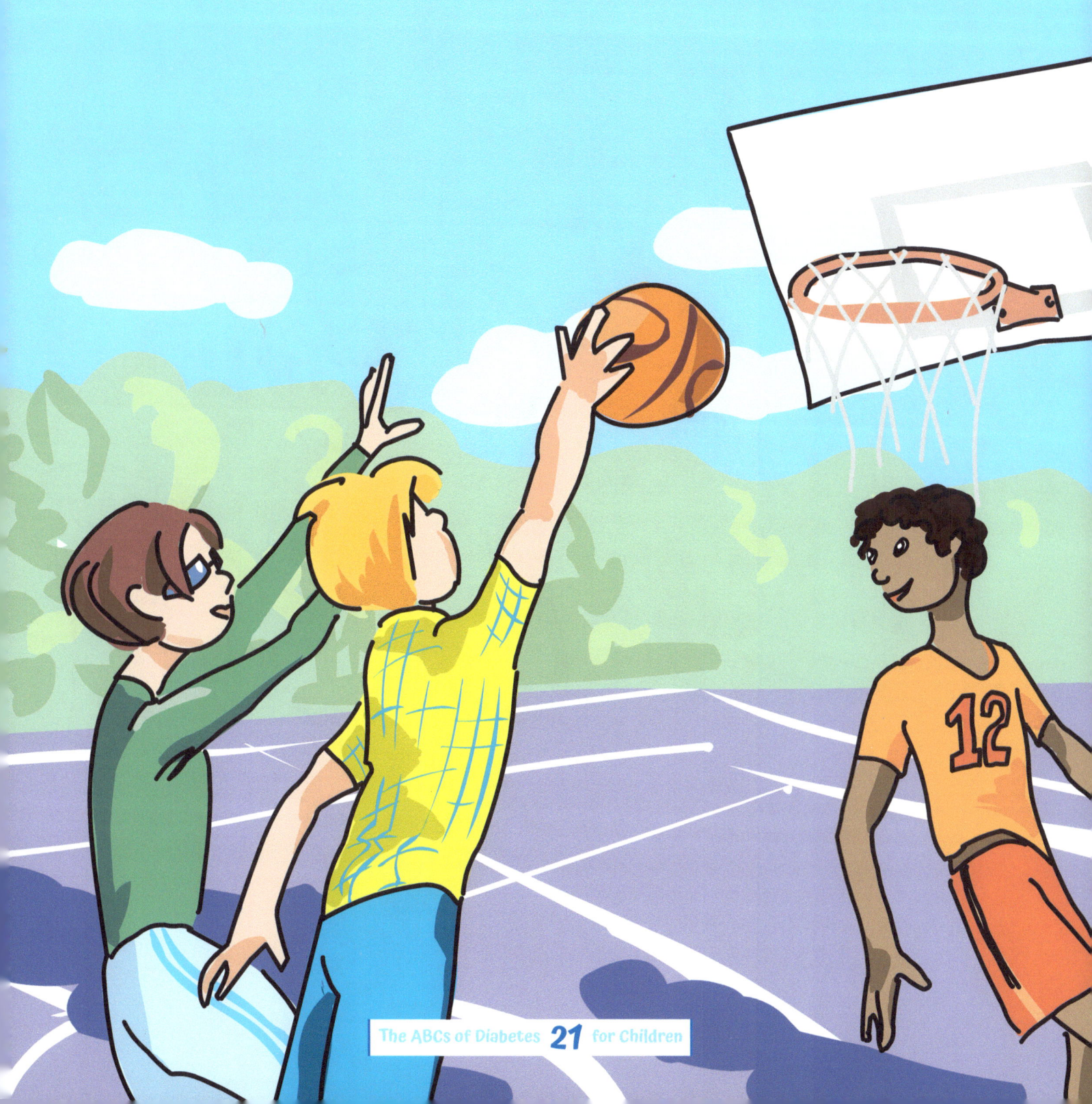

Because the insulin keys are not enough or not working well, INSULIN INJECTIONS will be given to get sugar into the cells.

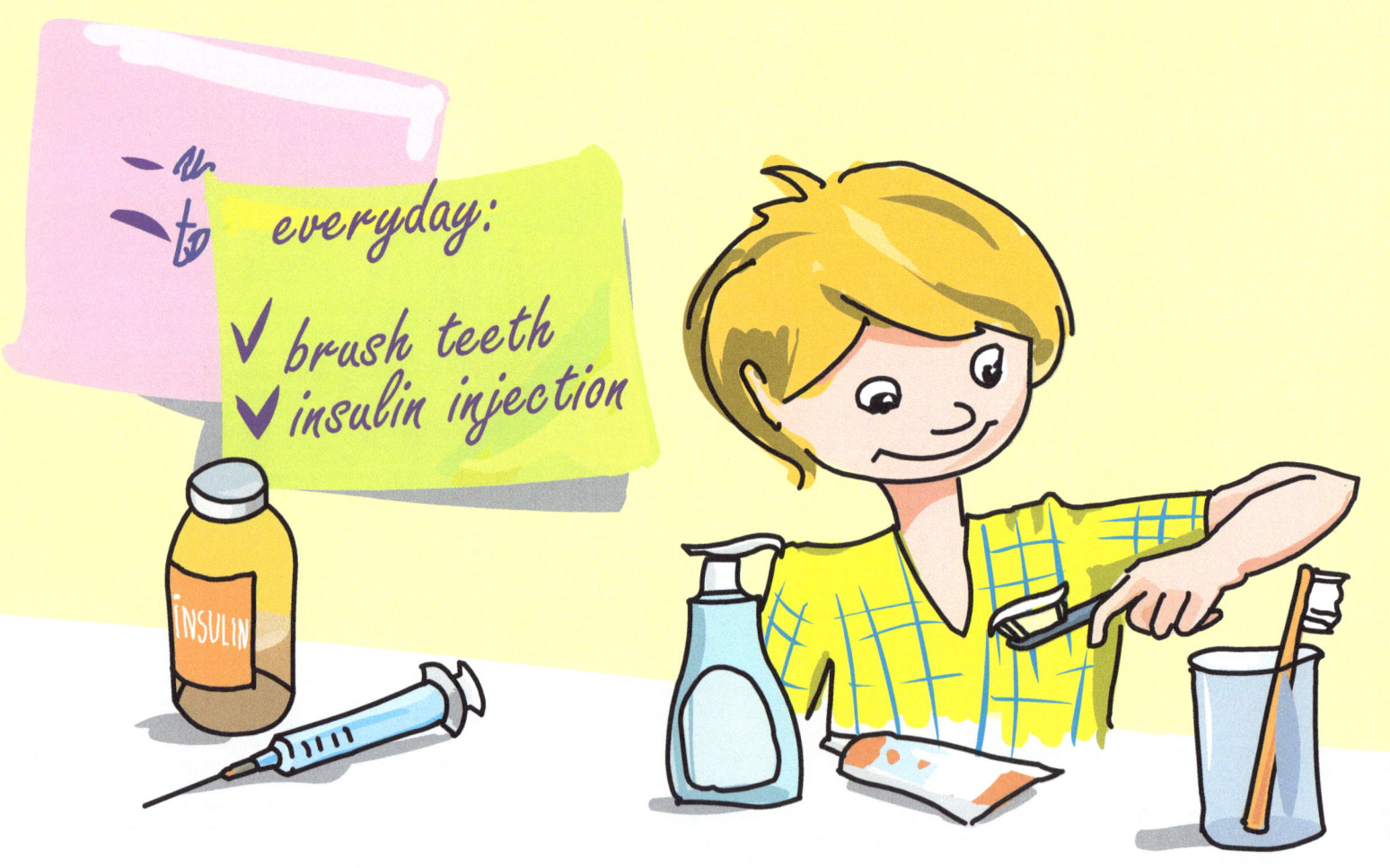

This procedure may hurt a bit,
But it is vital since the body can't work properly without it.

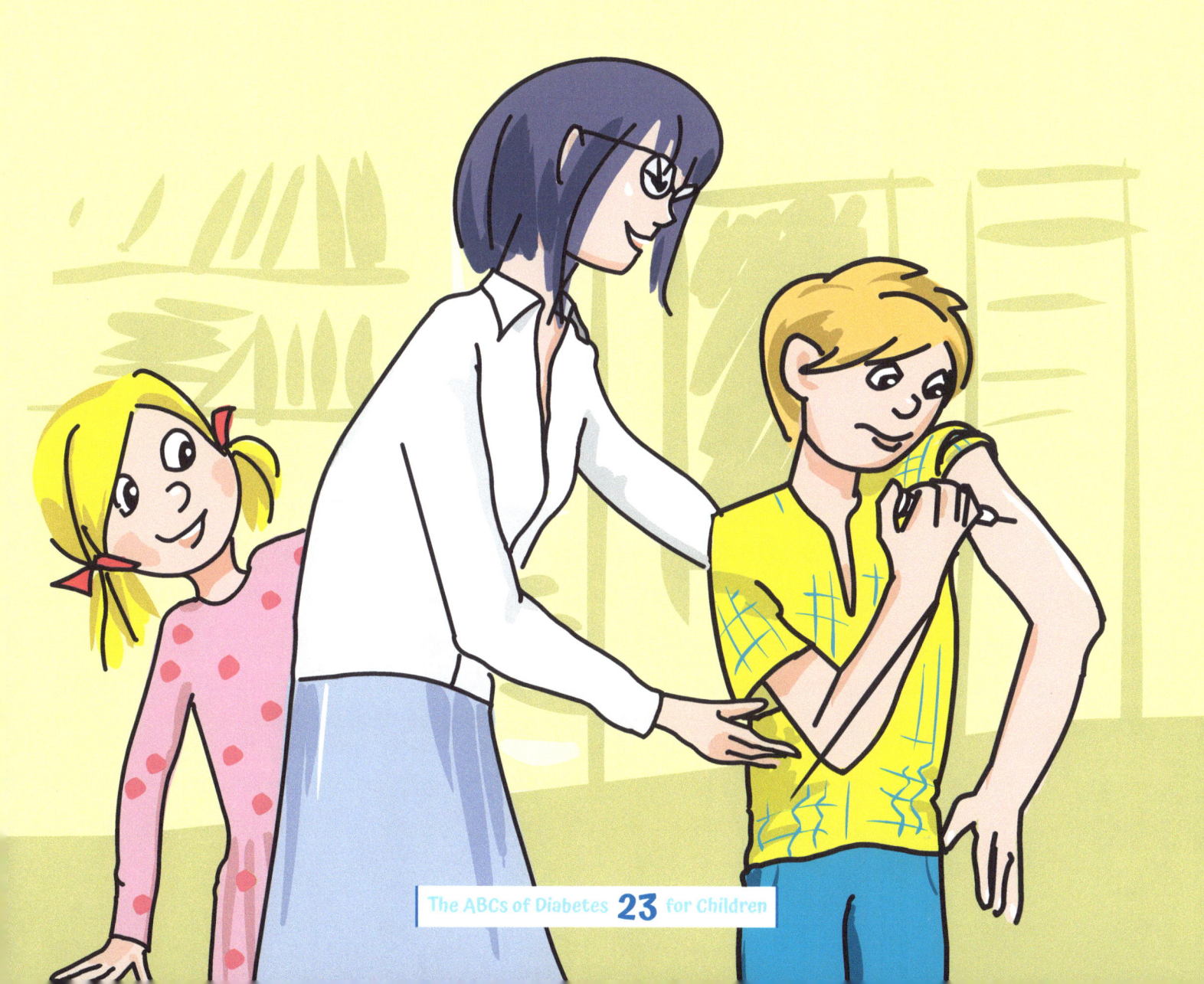

Blood sugar levels will be checked EVERYDAY.

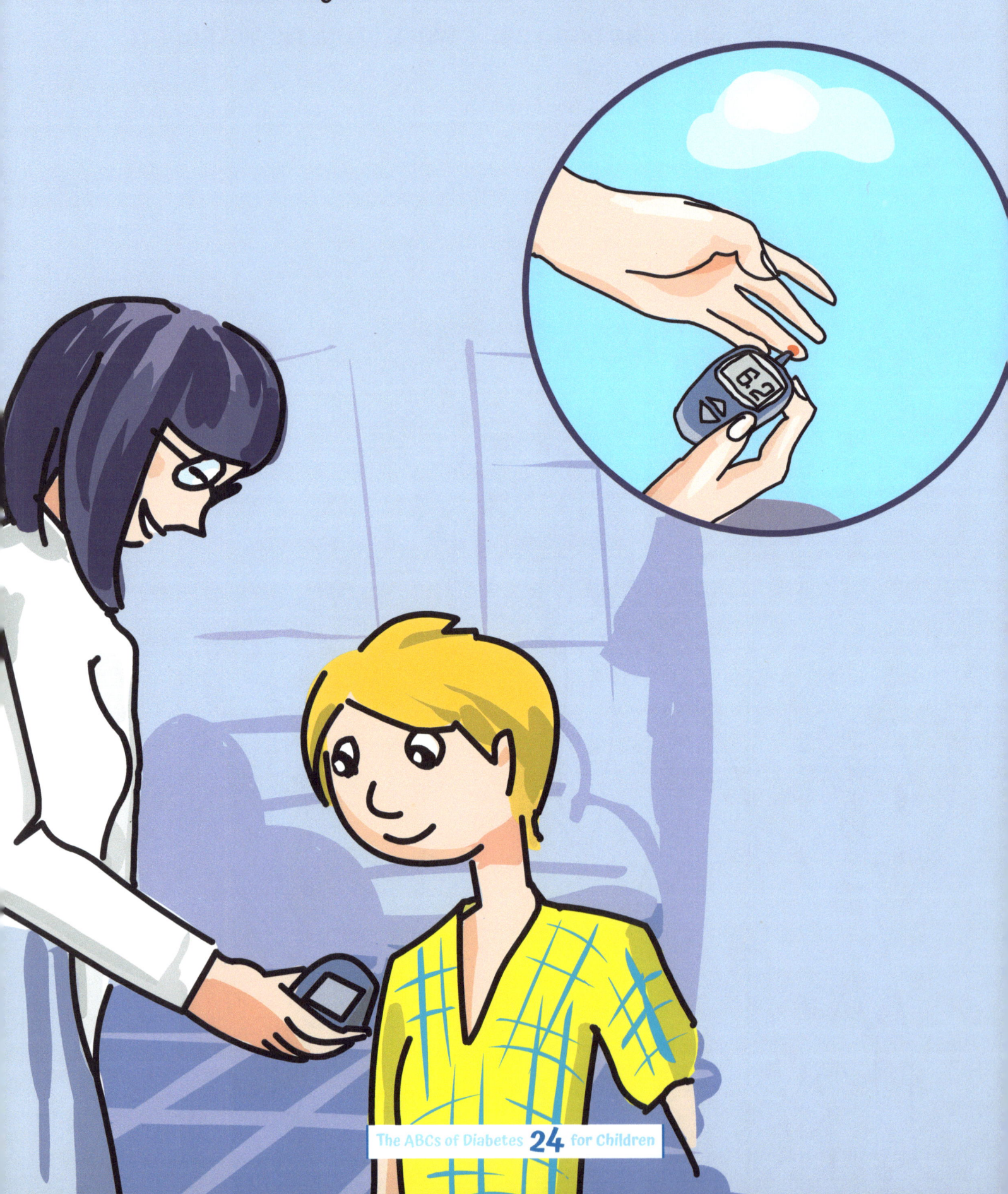

To make sure it is safe to RUN, SKIP, SWIM and PLAY.

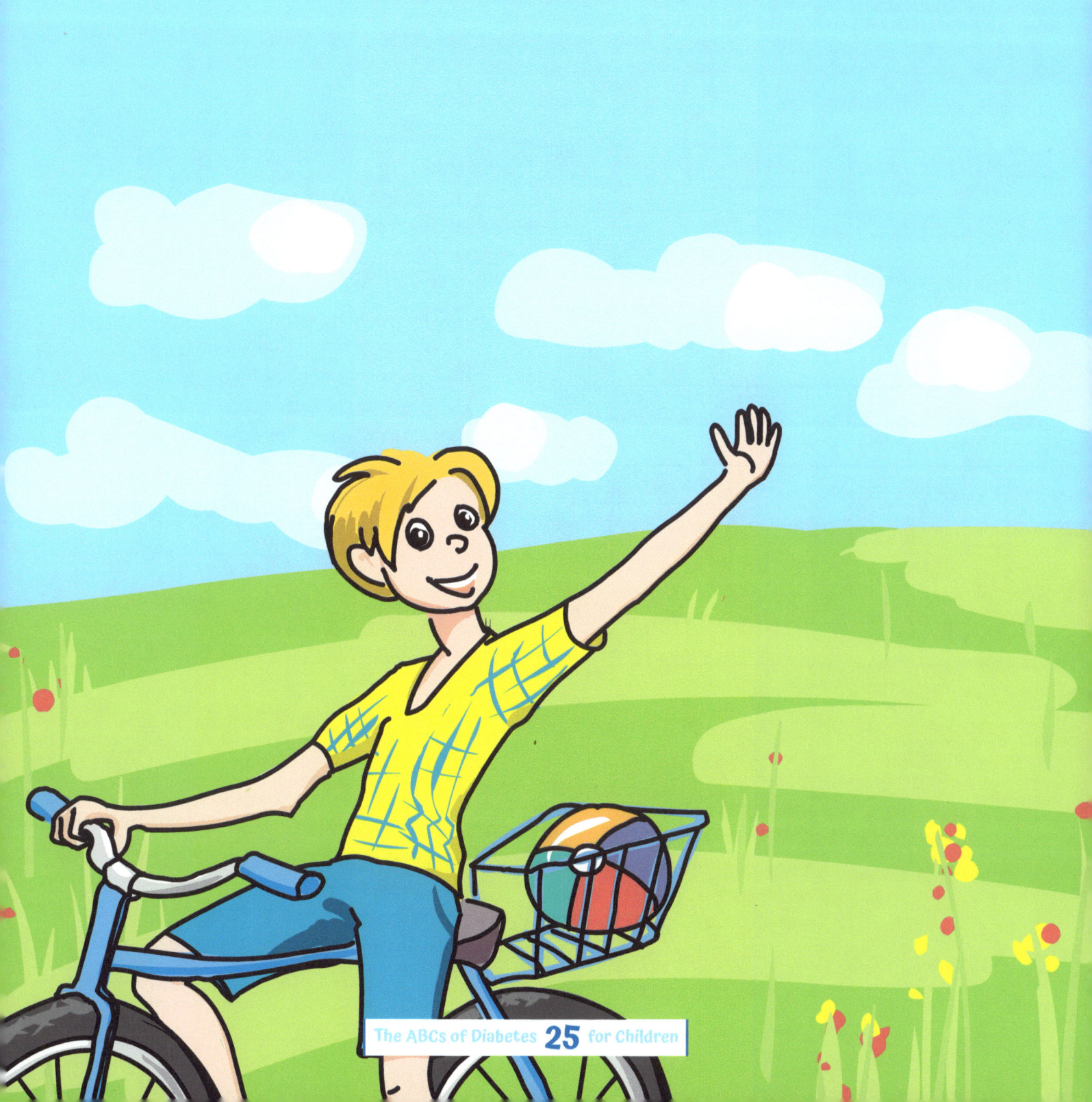

CROSSWORD PUZZLE
About Diabetes

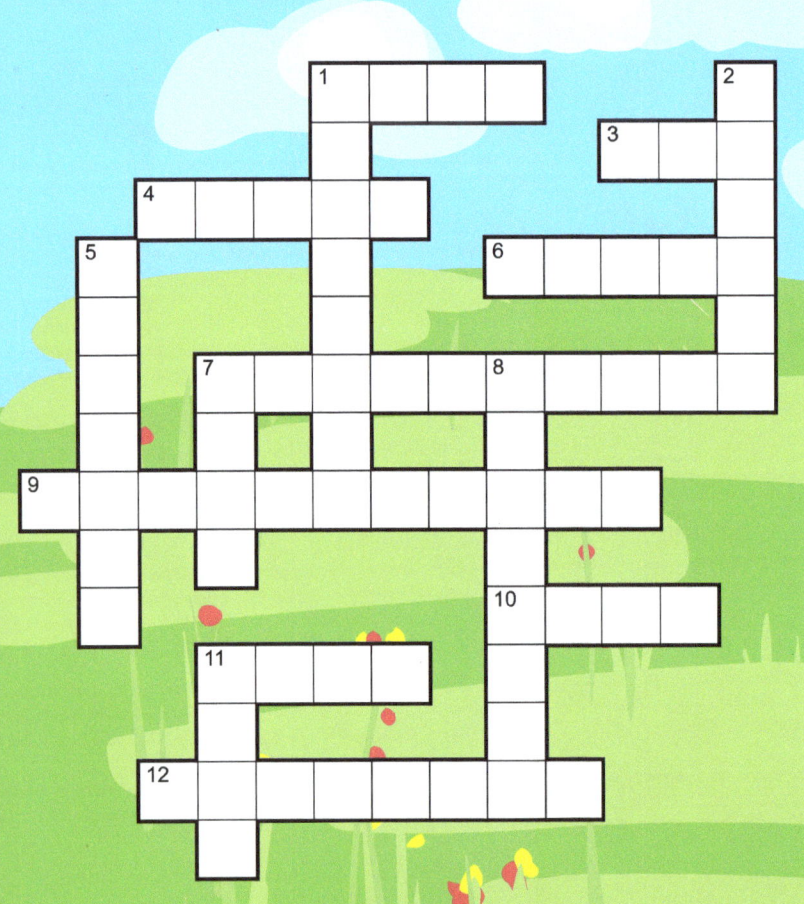

Across
1. Children do this often
3. Faster than walking
4. Fluid waste passed out through the kidneys
6. Used by the body for energy
7. Happening reguarly
9. Bloodflow through out the body
10. Very small part of the body
11. Movement in water
12. Occurs when the body can't use sugar normally

Down
1. Large gland, responsible for making insulin
2. The ability to be active
5. Your pancreas makes this
7. The things that people and animals eat
8. You should do this everyday
11. A rope must be used to do this

CROSSWORD PUZZLE
About Diabetes

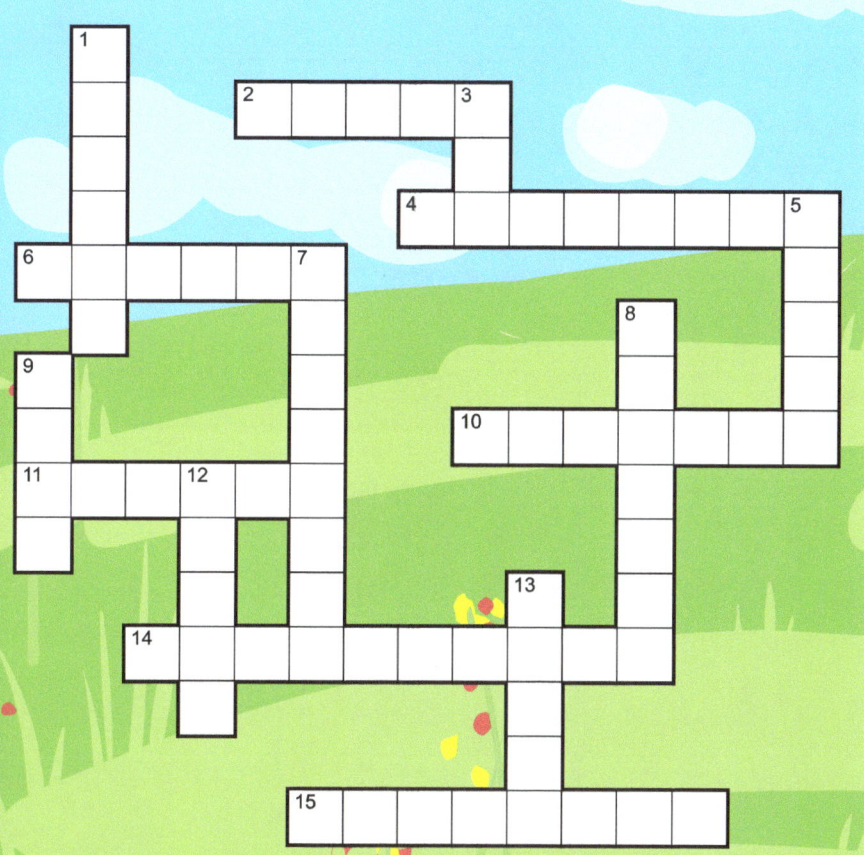

Across
2. Hit something with your knuckles
4. The ability to see
6. Produced by plants
10. When you are feeling for water
11. You visit this person when you are sick
14. Also produced by plants
15. More than one child is called

Down
1. Felt in your tummy when you need food
3. Used to open a lock
5. Your stomach or belly
7. An unexpected event
8. Father or mother
9. The physical self
12. You feel like this when you need rest
13. The heart pumps this throughout the body

WORD SEARCH PUZZLE
The ABCs of Diabetes Part 1

```
E D D F A T J M I I D L P V Q
H A Y L T N E U Q E R F Q V B
T B W M S M E I Y S Z Q B N B
K X R T T U O B Y I V N H G T
G D E N E R G Y E C O C O M R
X U O O C X X A O R O P M F F
D B L O O D S T R E A M I Q S
M G E O F M I U W X D V K E U
T A Q W P A N C R E A S T I R
U O T P I K S S E P N E O M O
H M W F Z W U F I L B I H V T
C E Z G I I L E A A L L R N C
P R L M W Q I U I Y F X E U V
C B B I E C N D K W Q U A D O
L F J E J G L K O V K C C G O
```

BLOODSTREAM
CELL
DIABETES
ENERGY
EXERCISE
FOOD
FREQUENTLY
INSULIN
PANCREAS
PLAY
RUN
SKIP
SUGAR
SWIM
URINE

WORD SEARCH PUZZLE
The ABCs of Diabetes Part 2

```
X U R N B R E K U T S B O D Y
R U A M T B P T P E X R E D T
O N Y G K G H U O H J R K O S
V L E Q Q N E R D L I H C Z R
O L U H D D B F A B L O O D I
X W N Q O C E D A Y R G N U H
G N R C C D N K P S P U K A T
D G S U T S E L B A T E G E V
A P U U O F G K Y Z R C Y X Y
N W J F R J Q A Q Q E E E U A
I A Y U C P D O F S S N N V Q
T H I M S D R W K I F A X T E
G T X D M S L I G E T Y Q O S
S H Y Q S U B H S T T M G U A
G X A S F N T I R E D F F F C
```

- BLOOD
- BODY
- CHILDREN
- DOCTOR
- EYESIGHT
- FRUITS
- HUNGRY
- KEY
- KNOCK
- PARENTS
- SURPRISE
- THIRSTY
- TIRED
- TUMMY
- VEGETABLES

CONTACT:

aj@poemsbyaj.com

www.poemsbyaj.com

/NurseJonesChat

/amandajohnjones

Amanda Jones

www.ingramcontent.com/pod-product-compliance
Lightning Source LLC
Chambersburg PA
CBHW051828210526
45473CB00005B/1781